Analytical Hypnotherapy

A Beginner's 3-Step Quick Start Guide, with an FAQ

copyright © 2023 Felicity Paulman

All rights reserved No part of this book may be reproduced, or stored in a retrieval system, or transmitted in any form or by any means, electronic, mechanical, photocopying, recording, or otherwise, without express written permission of the publisher.

Disclaimer

By reading this disclaimer, you are accepting the terms of the disclaimer in full. If you disagree with this disclaimer, please do not read the guide.

All of the content within this guide is provided for informational and educational purposes only, and should not be accepted as independent medical or other professional advice. The author is not a doctor, physician, nurse, mental health provider, or registered nutritionist/dietician. Therefore, using and reading this guide does not establish any form of a physician-patient relationship.

Always consult with a physician or another qualified health provider with any issues or questions you might have regarding any sort of medical condition. Do not ever disregard any qualified professional medical advice or delay seeking that advice because of anything you have read in this guide. The information in this guide is not intended to be any sort of medical advice and should not be used in lieu of any medical advice by a licensed and qualified medical professional.

The information in this guide has been compiled from a variety of known sources. However, the author cannot attest to or guarantee the accuracy of each source and thus should not be held liable for any errors or omissions.

You acknowledge that the publisher of this guide will not be held liable for any loss or damage of any kind incurred as a result of this guide or the reliance on any information provided within this guide. You acknowledge and agree that you assume all risk and responsibility for any action you undertake in response to the information in this guide.

Using this guide does not guarantee any particular result (e.g., weight loss or a cure). By reading this guide, you acknowledge that there are no guarantees to any specific outcome or results you can expect.

All product names, diet plans, or names used in this guide are for identification purposes only and are the property of their respective owners. The use of these names does not imply endorsement. All other trademarks cited herein are the property of their respective owners.

Where applicable, this guide is not intended to be a substitute for the original work of this diet plan and is, at most, a supplement to the original work for this diet plan and never a direct substitute. This guide is a personal expression of the facts of that diet plan.

Where applicable, persons shown in the cover images are stock photography models and the publisher has obtained the rights to use the images through license agreements with third-party stock image companies.

Table of Contents

Introduction   7
Background and History   9
   The Beginnings of Analytical Hypnotherapy   9
   The Influence of Other Therapies on Analytical Hypnotherapy   10
What Analytical Hypnotherapy Is All About   11
   How does it work?   12
Analytical Hypnotherapy Procedures   13
   What to expect in an Analytical Hypnotherapy?   14
Techniques Used in Hypnotherapy   18
Benefits of Analytical Hypnotherapy   22
Use Cases of Analytical Hypnotherapy   27
A Potential 3-Step Guide on How to Get Started with Analytical Hypnotherapy   35
   Step 1: Understand what Analytical Hypnotherapy is   35
   Step 2: Find a qualified therapist   36
   Step 3: Prepare for your session   37
Side Effects and Potential Risks of Analytical Hypnotherapy   38
Who Should Not Undergo Analytical Hypnotherapy?   44
Analytical Hypnotherapy vs. Psychoanalysis   48
Conclusion   51
FAQ About Analytical Hypnotherapy   53
References and Helpful Links   55

Introduction

Gaining insight into one's behavior is an invaluable skill. By reflecting on how one reacts in situations, it is possible to identify patterns, triggers, and thought processes that lead to particular reactions. Developing an understanding of what motivates these responses and the unhelpful habits associated with them can allow individuals to take steps toward changing them. Doing this enables a person to become aware of potentially detrimental reactions before they manifest, allowing for a conscious behavior change, or the adoption of more effective coping strategies. Analytical Hypnotherapy is an effective method for achieving this insight.

Analytical Hypnotherapy combines the use of hypnosis, psychodynamic techniques, and cognitive behavioral therapy to explore unconscious thought patterns and habits to bring them into conscious awareness. With such a tool at hand, those seeking to make significant changes in their lives can gain insight into the root causes of their difficulties and can learn to challenge ingrained beliefs and behaviors.

In this beginner's guide, we will tackle the following subtopics about Analytical Hypnotherapy:

- Background and history
- What is Analytical Hypnotherapy?
- How does it work?
- Analytical Hypnotherapy procedures
- What to expect in an Analytical Hypnotherapy?
- Techniques used in Analytical Hypnotherapy
- Benefits of Analytical Hypnotherapy
- Use cases of Analytical Hypnotherapy
- A potential 3-step guide on getting started with Analytical Hypnotherapy
- Side effects and potential risks of Analytical Hypnotherapy
- Who should not undergo Analytical Hypnotherapy?
- Analytical Hypnotherapy vs. Psychoanalysis

Keep reading to gain an understanding of Analytical Hypnotherapy and how it works, as well as a 3-step guide to help you get started with hypnoanalysis.

Background and History

The Beginnings of Analytical Hypnotherapy

Analytical hypnotherapy traces its roots back to 1841 when English doctor James Braid coined the term "hypnotism" as a way to describe what he believed was an altered state of consciousness. Around the same time, French neurologist Hippolyte Bernheim was practicing hypnotic suggestions to treat his patients' physical and mental ailments. Braid and Bernheim are credited with creating the base principles that would later be used in analytical hypnotherapy.

In 1950, American psychiatrist Milton H. Erickson revolutionized hypnotic therapy by introducing an informal conversational approach that focused on addressing client-specific therapeutic strategies that could be tailored to each patient's needs. In 1974, Theodore X. Barber introduced the term "cognitive-behavioral" which described how non-state theory could be applied to behavior therapy, paving the way for an even more effective form of analytical hypnotherapy to emerge in subsequent decades.

The Influence of Other Therapies on Analytical Hypnotherapy

Many cognitive and behavioral therapies were originally influenced by older hypnotherapeutic techniques like systematic desensitization—a technique derived from Lewis Wolberg's Medical Hypnosis (1948). Over time, these therapies have become more closely intertwined with analytical hypnotherapy as practitioners continue to develop new methods for treating psychological disorders using both traditional and modern approaches.

What Analytical Hypnotherapy Is All About

Analytical Hypnotherapy, also known as Hypnoanalysis is an approach to psychotherapy that combines hypnosis, psychoanalysis, and psychodynamic theories. It involves examining one's feelings and responses to uncover repressed traumas or unresolved conflicts in the subconscious.

Analytical Hypnotherapy is a collaborative process between the client and a licensed hypnotherapist, in which the goal is to explore underlying causes of psychological distress stemming from physical, emotional, mental, or spiritual sources. The therapist guides the client through a trance-like state to reach suppressed memories, thoughts, and emotions that are out of conscious awareness.

The primary goal of Analytical Hypnotherapy is to provide a resolution for any underlying issues or hidden beliefs that may exist. It seeks to equip individuals with strategies they can use both during and after their sessions to effectively manage their condition. Additionally, it encourages self-reflection and personal growth which can result in improved emotional well-being overall.

How does it work?

Hypnoanalysis is a form of therapy focused on hypnosis-induced regression, which is intended to uncover the underlying psychological cause of a person's distress. This meta-theoretical approach views certain issues as having a hidden origin or early trauma that may be causing current symptoms.

In practice, the therapist begins by hypnotizing the patient and then guiding them through memories to bring out the mental aspects behind their challenge. It is theorized that once these issues are identified, further treatment can target them directly for a resolution. Thus, hypnoanalysis is one way among many for psychiatrists and other providers to help clients pursue deeper exploration and understanding of their mental health conditions.

Analytical Hypnotherapy Procedures

Analytical Hypnotherapy is a subset of psychological treatment that utilizes hypnosis as a tool to better comprehend and treat the fundamental problems at the core of a client's condition. Through the use of guided imagery, the therapist assists the patient in entering a state of relaxation as the first step toward reaching this level. To do this, the person must first fall into a state of profound relaxation. This allows them to become more receptive to ideas and allows them to investigate their unconscious brains.

The therapist will utilize verbal or memory clues as the session proceeds to assist the patient in accessing deeper layers of understanding about themselves and the experiences they have had. Doing this may allow them to find dynamics inside themselves that lead to their unconscious behavior, and as a result, it can help them to work through any tensions that are making it difficult for them to go ahead in life.

To aid in the investigation of a patient's thoughts and feelings, the therapist may also depend on a range of various strategies.

It is possible to obtain a deeper understanding of the patient's underlying ideas and experiences by including metaphor, narrative or visualizing those experiences as part of a therapy session. During this in-depth analysis, therapists have the opportunity to obtain useful knowledge that may be used to supplement the findings of other lines of inquiry and offer beneficial illumination as they work with their clients.

What to expect in an Analytical Hypnotherapy?

In general, the following are some of the things that you might anticipate feeling or experiencing throughout an analytical hypnotherapy session:

1. The therapist will ask you questions about your medical history and the nature of your problem.

During an analytical hypnotherapy session, the therapist will often question you about your medical history as well as the nature of the issue that you are experiencing. It is possible to identify and shed light on the underlying feelings and triggers that are the source of the difficulties that are now being presented via the use of this well-structured discourse. This enables possibilities to link dispersed thoughts, allowing exploration of fresh views as well as significant reflections on prior experiences. The session is generally marked by remarks that are both insightful and thought-provoking.

2. The therapist will then explain what analytical hypnotherapy is and how it can help you.

Anyone interested in seeing larger effects from other forms of therapy may find that participating in an analytical hypnotherapy session is an instructive and beneficial experience. Before commencing the practice of hypnotherapy, the therapist will often begin by providing some early instruction concerning hypnotherapy. This may involve orienting clients as to what hypnotherapy is, how it works, and how it may help them attain their objectives related to emotional well-being.

Hypnotherapy is effective in helping people achieve their goals connected to emotional well-being. The clients of this kind of psychotherapy may anticipate a serene and trustworthy environment during their sessions, during which a thorough evaluation of their psychological well-being and emotional condition will take place.

3. The therapist will then induce a state of hypnosis.

Your therapist will lead you on a personal journey of emotional discovery as part of an analytical hypnotherapy session. This trip will be led by your therapist. During the session, relaxation and hypnosis are utilized to zero in on certain situations and experiences to isolate the fundamental factors that contribute to misery. Your ability to judge is temporarily halted, and you get access to levels of consciousness that you may have lost or neglected in the past.

4. After the session, the therapist will discuss their findings with you.

Following the conclusion of the session, your therapist will talk to you about the findings of the session. This can be a beneficial experience for both parties because it allows the therapist to further explain what was discovered during the hypnotherapy process and gives the client the chance to ask additional questions or reflect on any insights that may have come up as a result of the hypnotherapy session. It is essential to take the time to focus on these findings because they may give great insight into habits and emotions that may help to influence your present and future. Taking the time to reflect on these findings could provide valuable information.

5. Treatment usually consists of several sessions.

The treatment for analytical hypnotherapy is often broken up over several different sessions as it is a process. The therapist may discuss a variety of topics during each session based on what emerges from the discussions that took place in the sessions that came before. When patients feel more at ease with the relationship that exists between themselves and their therapists, they frequently discover that they make better strides toward their treatment goals and can explore more profound feelings with more ease. In the end, the practice of analytical hypnotherapy can deliver a one-of-a-kind and life-changing encounter that ultimately results in increased emotional mastery.

In general, analytic hypnotherapy has the potential to be an extremely useful technique for assisting individuals in gaining insight into themselves and the fundamental nature of their problems. This sort of therapy has the potential to be very helpful in assisting with the creation of good and long-lasting change when it is approached with due deliberation and guided by an experienced therapist.

Techniques Used in Hypnotherapy

Hypnotherapy is a method that is used to induce a trance, but hypnoanalysis gives the therapist the ability to evaluate how patterns that were created in the patient's history may be contributing to the patient's current issues. The following are some of the methods that are utilized in hypnotherapy to conduct in-depth investigations to acquire access to conflicts that are stored inside the unconscious mind.

Relaxation

The initial stage in hypnotherapy is to assist the patient in achieving a state of relaxation. This can be accomplished via the use of several different techniques, such as slow, deep breathing, gradual muscle relaxation, or guided visualization. After the patient has been made comfortable, the therapist can start to work on producing a hypnotic state in the patient.

Focusing on a Single Point

Directing the client's attention to a single point is one of the most popular ways used to induce hypnosis. It is possible to do this by directing the client's gaze toward a stationary item, such as a pencil or a certain area on the wall. After that, the therapist will start counting backward from 100, being sure to say each number slowly and clearly as they go along. As the client continues to concentrate on the item while listening to the therapist count backward, they will begin to experience a sense of relaxation and their mind will become more receptive to the therapist's ideas.

Eye Fixation

Eye Fixation is another prominent method that is used to induce hypnosis, and its name comes from the practice itself. In this technique, the subject is instructed to concentrate their attention on a revolving item, such as a swinging watch or a flickering candle flame. The longer the customer focuses on the object, the more calm and receptive their mind will become to the customer's ideas.

Arm Levitation

Arm Levitation is one of the most well-known methods that may be employed in hypnosis, and it's also one of the most effective. To do this, the client will need to be seated in a chair and instructed to keep their arms by their sides. The client will then be instructed by the therapist to imagine that as time passes, their arms become lighter and lighter until they ultimately float up into the air. When the client concentrates on the picture, their mind will become more open to the hypnotist's recommendations, and they may find themselves drifting off into a hypnotic state.

Visual Imagery

Hypnosis also frequently makes use of a method known as "visual imagery," which involves the participant imagining things. In this technique, the client is instructed to close their eyes and see themselves in a calm or soothing situation, such as lazing about on a beach or floating in a pool. When the client concentrates on the picture, their mind will become more open to the hypnotist's recommendations, and they may find themselves drifting off into a hypnotic state.

Auditory Imaging

Auditory imagery is quite similar to visual imagery; however, instead of envisioning visuals in their head, the client concentrates on soothing sounds or music during this phase of the process. This can be accomplished by giving the client audio relaxation exercises or guided meditations to listen to as they work on themselves. The client's mind will become more sensitive to suggestions as they listen to these exercises and envision calming sounds or music, and as a result, they may enter a state of hypnosis at some point throughout the session.

Kinesthetic Imagery

Kinesthetic imagery is another type of visual imagery that involves imagining oneself experiencing the physical sensations of relaxation, such as floating on a cloud or sinking into a soft mattress. Kinesthetic imagery is a form of guided imagery that can be used to treat a variety of mental and physical conditions. The more the client concentrates on these pictures and imagines himself feeling these sensations, the more open their mind will become to suggestions, and the more likely it is that they will enter a state of hypnosis.

After the client has reached a state of hypnosis, the therapist can then proceed to investigate the client's unconscious mind and treat any underlying issues or conflicts that could be present.

Benefits of Analytical Hypnotherapy

Hypnotherapy is associated with a wide variety of positive effects. The following are some of the most widespread ones:

1. Hypnotherapy is effective in treating a wide range of disorders and ailments.

Hypnotherapy is a type of psychotherapy that focuses on the unconscious part of the mind and has been practiced for a considerable amount of time. It is a helpful method for tackling psychological and emotional concerns, such as managing chronic pain and overcoming a phobia of flying, for example.

Over the years, it has garnered support as a method supported by evidence for the treatment of a wide variety of diseases, ranging from severe depression to addiction problems. Studies have indicated that the therapeutic approach that it takes can be useful in treating illnesses such as eating disorders, post-traumatic stress disorder (PTSD), smoking cessation, and even lowering nightmares in children.

This might be because hypnotherapy is capable of putting the patient into a calm state, which is required for accessing important cognitive regions and assisting the patient in gaining a deeper understanding of how their moods influence their day-to-day existence. Overall, hypnotherapy is highly helpful in treating a variety of diseases that call for attention related to mental health, and it should be incorporated as part of an extensive treatment plan because of this.

2. Hypnotherapy is a therapeutic option that is both risk-free and effective.

Hypnotherapy is a sort of psychological treatment that is both risk-free and increasingly common, and its popularity has been growing steadily over the past few decades. It is utilized by psychotherapists who are both trained and experienced to assist patients in overcoming a broad variety of challenges, including but not limited to anxiety, phobias, addiction, and depression. It is successful because it can penetrate the subconscious and treat the underlying mental processes that may be the source of the discomfort or suffering.

Hypnotherapy assists the patient in reaching a concentrated state, which might offer the clarity that is required to recognize the patient's issues and begin working to resolve them. In addition to being risk-free, hypnotherapy is particularly useful for altering deeply ingrained patterns of behavior. This allows an individual to make changes that are significant to them and that endure throughout their lifetime.

3. Hypnotherapy can be used in conjunction with other forms of treatment as an adjunctive therapy.

It has been shown that combining hypnotherapy with other forms of treatment produces excellent results in resolving issues such as pain management and substance abuse. Hypnotherapy may even prove useful as an adjunct in the treatment of mental health conditions such as post-traumatic stress disorder. Individuals might anticipate more favorable results from their course of therapy if they incorporate hypnotherapy into their tailored treatment plans and give it serious consideration.

4. Patients can have a greater sense of control through the use of hypnotherapy.

Hypnotherapy is an intriguing and powerful sort of therapy that may be a terrific method to help individuals acquire control over challenging habits or ideas. It can also be a great way to help people relax and enjoy the therapeutic process. It has the potential to have a significant impact on the transformation of self-use difficulties such as addiction, depression, or anxiety when it is done appropriately.

Patients are guided into a hypnotic trance with the assistance of hypnotherapy, which then bestows upon them the ability to exercise control over their identities, thereby assisting them in developing a deeper comprehension of who they are and easing them into a state more conducive to relaxation and transformation. As the patient reaches this profoundly changed state of consciousness and as various patterns are deployed to trigger positive behavior changes, the patient becomes empowered to think positively and, eventually, to make the required behavioral alterations that they wish.

The end effect is frequently an improvement in well-being across a variety of domains, including relationships, productivity at work, or physical health. It should come as no surprise that hypnosis has grown in popularity not just among therapists but also among the people they treat.

5. The use of hypnotherapy can contribute to improved outcomes for patients.

Hypnotherapy is proven to be a useful tool for improving patient outcomes, and there has been an uptick in the field of medicine interested in utilizing it. It is possible to successfully treat a wide variety of physical and mental disorders by making use of hypnotic techniques, such as guided imagery and exercises that emphasize concentrated breathing.

It has been shown that hypnosis can give individuals improved coping abilities, particularly when it comes to dealing with pain and anxiety. In addition, hypnosis has the potential to be more effective than other forms of therapy in helping patients kick undesirable habits like nail biting and smoking. It should come as no surprise that hypnosis is becoming increasingly popular as an essential component of holistic health care given the significant advantages that it offers.

Use Cases of Analytical Hypnotherapy

Analytical hypnotherapy is effective for a large number of patients; it has been utilized to treat a wide variety of diseases, including depression, anxiety, phobias, stress management, and recovery from addiction, amongst others.

Anxiety

For people looking for successful treatment for anxiety, hypnoanalysis might be a useful therapeutic strategy to utilize. It is possible to enter the subconscious mind and investigate the underlying reasons for anxiety by using this method. This enables the individual to fully tackle the difficulties that have been brewing below the surface for some time. Consequently, those who opt to undergo hypnoanalysis uncover hitherto unknown strategies for coping with their fears, allowing them to start living a life that is both happier and more alleviated.

Depression

Hypnoanalysis is a novel method of treating depression that differs from other approaches in that it helps patients gain insight into the underlying factors that contribute to the development of depressive symptoms. Hypnosis is a technique that may be utilized by trained experts to assist depressed persons in gaining insight into the events and emotions that have played a significant role in the development of their condition and in gaining access to novel coping mechanisms.

People are encouraged to communicate their sentiments and take control of how they think and feel about their mental health difficulties while undergoing hypnoanalysis. This method of treatment has frequently been shown to be quite effective in easing the suffering caused by depression in patients while simultaneously assisting them in gaining knowledge of and confidence in their ability to manage the feelings that accompany the condition.

Addiction

Hypnoanalysis is a method of psychotherapy that combines the use of hypnosis with standard talk therapy to assist with addressing issues that are more deeply rooted. Hypnoanalysis is often used to treat addiction. The goal of hypnoanalysis practitioners is to assist their clients in changing their habits and achieving long-term success by focusing on the resolution of traumatic experiences and unpleasant memories.

Since of this, it is particularly well-suited for the treatment of addiction because it may address problematic habits and give skills like visualization and cognitive reframing that can act as effective approaches for preventing relapse. In addition, although talk therapy by itself may be effective in treating addiction, research has shown that combining it with hypnosis significantly increases the success rate. This is possible because hypnosis can tap into a person's subconscious motivations in a way that traditional talk therapy cannot.

PTSD

Hypnoanalysis is a strategy that can be helpful in the treatment of post-traumatic stress disorder (PTSD). This is due to hypnoanalysis's capacity to investigate memories and feelings that are stored in the subconscious mind. In hypnoanalysis, hypnotic procedures such as guided imagery and trance induction are used to create a state of heightened suggestibility in the client.

This state enables the therapist to access the client's internal frame of reference, making it possible for formerly hidden or suppressed thought patterns to be brought to the client's attention for conscious analysis. Individuals who suffer from PTSD can work with their traumatic experiences in a way that is efficient and successful without having to spend months participating in psychotherapy sessions. This is accomplished by directly attacking unfulfilled psychological hurdles.

These results have the potential to give vital insights into how individuals perceive and react to traumatic experiences, which are issues that need to be addressed before any substantial improvements can take place. Because of this, hypnoanalysis is a fantastic choice for everyone who wants to work with the things that have happened to them and go on with their lives in a healthy way.

Anger Management

Hypnoanalysis is beginning to acquire respect for its potential to help individuals better regulate their emotions, particularly anger. One area in which this skill is being utilized is anger management. People can get insight into the root of their emotional discomfort and learn relaxation skills that can help them stay in control when confronted with tough situations via the use of this sort of treatment. They will be able to build healthier reactions to emotional stimuli and make more rational judgments in the heat of the moment if they work on enhancing their self-awareness.

People can achieve a more peaceful state of mind and have more fulfilling exchanges with one another as a direct result of this. In addition, this method of treatment is very useful for people who frequently find themselves being overburdened by demanding circumstances or emotional responses that they struggle to keep under control on their own.

Phobias

The use of hypnoanalysis as a strategy for the treatment of phobias is becoming increasingly popular. This evidence-based strategy is helping individuals to handle their fear of flying and public speaking in a manner that is more holistic by employing calming mantras and guided visualizations.

During the process of hypnoanalysis, which is also known as hypnotherapy, an individual collaborates with a practitioner who has received professional training to investigate the underlying causes of their phobias. At the same time, the individual is guided into a state of heightened awareness and relaxation that enables them to rethink and reevaluate their feelings regarding the experience. The method is an efficient means of overcoming anxieties that would have been impossible to conquer in any other way.

Sleep Disorders

Hypnoanalysis is becoming an increasingly well-liked kind of treatment for people who have trouble getting sufficient amounts of restful sleep. Sleep problems can benefit from hypnoanalysis. Hypnosis is utilized in this kind of treatment to reframe and reprogram a person's behaviors, cognitions, and attitudes, all of which may be contributing factors to the individual's inability to get the necessary amount of sleep. This medication also helps to alleviate any accompanying worry or tension, which is commonly a side effect of insomnia as well as other sleep problems that are connected.

Individuals can make good adjustments in their day-to-day routines while steadily increasing their overall quality of sleep by engaging with a competent hypnotist who can guide them through the hypnosis process. Hypnoanalysis is a method that is both risk-free and non-invasive, and it may be of use to everyone who wants to increase the amount of sleep they get or the quality of it.

Pain Management

Hypnoanalysis has been utilized for many years to assist those who endure constant pain in becoming more accustomed to their circumstances. This psychological approach has the potential to be an effective therapeutic option that can lessen the intensity of chronic pain as well as the associated misery. Individuals are instructed to direct their attention inside during periods of pain and to engage in self-hypnosis to lessen the severity of the pain and any potential factors that may be producing it.

Therefore, hypnoanalysis can not only assist in the management of pain in the here and now, but it can also function as a preventative treatment for pain in the future by helping an individual understand what causes them to experience discomfort. This strategy can help people develop higher awareness and comprehension of their body via alert meditation, which can then be used to assist them in the continuous fight against their physical ailments.

Weight Loss

Hypnoanalysis has become a more acceptable method for addressing harmful habits connected to weight loss and well-being. Hypnoanalysis can help people lose weight. The client is put into a calm condition and permitted to reach their subconscious during the procedure.

Once there, they can recognize and alter behaviors that may be causing them to gain weight or preventing them from losing it. Instead of focusing on short-term fixes such as going on a diet or avoiding particular foods, clients may find out what is driving their urge for unhealthy behaviors with the assistance of the process, which helps get to the bottom of the problem.

Clients are also able to make the progressive lifestyle modifications necessary for lasting health advantages when the underlying issues that are causing their health problems are uncovered. In the end, hypnoanalysis provides an effective approach for tackling food-related habits that have historically been difficult to regulate. These behaviors include binge eating and compulsive overeating.

However, in general, this kind of therapy may help improve emotional well-being by resolving any underlying difficulties or hidden beliefs that may be present. The possible advantages vary depending on the requirements of each individual, but in general, this form of treatment can help enhance emotional well-being.

A Potential 3-Step Guide on How to Get Started with Analytical Hypnotherapy

The following instructions might assist you in getting started with hypnoanalysis as a viable treatment option if you are interested in doing so:

Step 1: Understand what Analytical Hypnotherapy is

It has been demonstrated that analytical hypnotherapy is an effective method for treating a variety of psychological conditions. Hypnosis and reframing are two strong strategies that may be utilized to get access to the underlying reasons for one's misery. This style of treatment makes use of both of these tools.

Analytical hypnotherapy is a type of hypnotherapy that helps patients discover and investigate the underlying causes of their problems so that they may make good changes in their lives. This is accomplished using a combination of trance work, talking, and relaxation methods. Before beginning this sort of therapy, one has to have a solid comprehension of how it treats patients to get the most favorable results.

Step 2: Find a qualified therapist

If you are thinking about giving analytical hypnotherapy a shot, the first thing you need to do is locate a therapist who is properly trained to perform the technique. Try to find a therapist who has been awarded a certificate of completion from either the American Society of Clinical Hypnosis or the British Society of Clinical Hypnosis. You might also try contacting the mental health association in your region, or you could search online for therapists in the vicinity of where you live.

When it comes to acquiring the appropriate Analytical Hypnotherapy treatment, one of the most important tasks is researching potential therapists and learning about their credentials. Taking the time to investigate individual skills, license criteria, patient reviews, and price information may all be beneficial in the search for an appropriate practitioner.

It is also a good idea to investigate any therapeutic tools they employ, such as books or movies that may be suggested, however, the extent to which you do this will depend on the amount of ease you are seeking. You will be better able to make an educated selection and feel more confident in your choice of qualified therapy providers if you do sufficient research before making your pick.

Step 3: Prepare for your session

Preparing yourself for your appointment with your therapist is the third step in getting started with analytical hypnotherapy (Analytical Hypnotherapy). If you do this, both you and the therapist will be able to make the most of each session, which will result in a more positive and productive experience overall. This preparation can be made in several different ways. It might require conducting research on the subject or asking your contemporaries for specific information about it.

In addition, keeping notes both before and after sessions enables you to monitor your development and pinpoint any areas in which either your knowledge or the effectiveness of the therapy is lacking. Finally, it is important to discuss your sentiments about the process in advance, regardless of whether those feelings are pleasant or bad. Doing so ensures that both you and the therapist are fully prepared for what is to come.

Hypnotherapy that uses an analytical approach can be an effective method for resolving any psychological problems that may be present. If you use this kind of treatment and follow these three steps, you will be well on your way to attaining the result you want from using it. Analytical hypnotherapy is an effective option that can have long-lasting positive effects on one's health. This technique requires both knowledge and patience.

Side Effects and Potential Risks of Analytical Hypnotherapy

Although it has the potential to be a useful therapeutic tool, analytical hypnotherapy is not without its associated hazards. The following is a list of some of the potential hazards and adverse effects that may occur either during or after a session:

1. Analytical hypnotherapy is not supported by sufficient data from the scientific community to be considered effective.

Analytical hypnotherapy is a form of therapy that makes extensive use of hypnosis as its primary method of treatment. Its proponents assert that it may discover the underlying causes of psychological problems and bring to light memories and ideas that are kept hidden from conscious awareness. Even though this condition-specific approach shows promise for people who are looking for relief from the troubling mental health issues they are experiencing, scientific research has not yet been conducted to support these claims.

As a result, the efficacy and authenticity of analytical hypnotherapy are both in question. Although there have been some preliminary studies that show that reducing 'dissociations' brought about by the trance state may assist in the treatment of some symptoms, further study is required before any conclusions can be drawn on the effectiveness of this kind of treatment. The only proof that analytical hypnotherapy is effective that we have at our disposal at this time is anecdotal.

2. The use of analytical hypnotherapy is not backed by sufficient data from the scientific community to suggest that it is safe.

Analytical hypnotherapy has been used for a long time as a method for determining the underlying causes of symptoms and diseases; however, the practice's application has recently come under investigation due to a lack of scientific proof. There is no doubt that analytical hypnotherapy has been successful for some patients; nevertheless, because there is a lack of sufficient scientific data defining how and why it works, there is substantial worry about how safe it is.

Even though there is empirical evidence to suggest that the method is efficient, further study has to be carried out to achieve a deeper comprehension not only of the method's efficiency but also of the inherent safety measures that it entails. When taking into consideration analytical hypnotherapy as a potential treatment option, we need to exercise extreme caution until more study has been conducted and the results published.

3. The use of analytical hypnotherapy might not be successful for all patients.

Analytical hypnotherapy may have helped many people in the past, but it is not effective for everyone. There are numerous success stories from individuals who have profited from it. When a person is in a condition similar to a trance, they may have trouble identifying or articulating certain ideas or feelings. This may be the reason for this phenomenon.

However, some therapists believe that analytical hypnotherapy should still be considered an option that should be explored, even though it is not effective for everyone. According to these therapists, the success of analytical hypnotherapy is still largely dependent on the expertise and dedication of the therapist managing a patient's sessions.

4. Headaches, dizziness, and nausea are some of the possible adverse reactions that might result after undergoing analytical hypnotherapy.

The use of analytical hypnotherapy, which falls under the categories of alternative and complementary treatment, has the potential to offer considerable advantages to patients' mental health. Unfortuitously, it has been linked to a few unpleasant side effects, such as nausea, dizziness, and headaches. According to some reports, the primary reason for this is the degree of intense attention that is required for the procedure.

This level of concentration might be overwhelming for those who are not accustomed to being in such a state of awareness. Individuals who are receiving analytical hypnotherapy should adhere to the instructions given to them by their doctor and give their bodies adequate time to adapt if this is required. It is essential that anybody interested in attempting this form of treatment first consult with a qualified specialist who can provide suitable direction and oversight.

5. Analytical hypnotherapy has been shown to induce undesirable feelings in patients, including dread and anxiety in some cases.

Analytical hypnotherapy has the potential to be a useful method of treating a variety of mental health conditions; yet, it also has the potential to cause patients to feel a range of unpleasant emotions, including dread and anxiety. For example, people may experience anxiety when they are forced to relive unpleasant experiences from their past.

Before deciding on treatment, it is essential for patients who are considering analytical hypnotherapy to have a conversation with their therapist about the possibility of feeling dread or anxiety as a result of the treatment. Analytical hypnotherapy can still be an effective treatment option for those coping with a variety of problems, provided that enough preparation and care are taken.

6. Some people report that analytical hypnotherapy makes them re-experience terrible memories.

Patients are encouraged to discover connections and investigate deeper implications between their past experiences and the way they behave in the current day during their treatment sessions. Unfortuitously, an individual may be forced to revisit terrible experiences as a result of analytical hypnotherapy.

It is not unheard of for clients who are in a hypnotic state to regress to unpleasant memories, which then leads the therapist to acquire an understanding of what traumatic experiences may have triggered the initial symptoms. Consequently, individuals who participate in these sessions to reevaluate their lives should be informed that there is a risk that they will be forced to relive distressing experiences from their past.

7. There is a possibility that analytical hypnotherapy will conflict with the other medical therapies that you are doing.

Analytical hypnotherapy, like any other form of medical treatment, requires patients to be aware of the possibility that it could interact negatively with the other forms of medical care they are currently getting. Hypnosis, for instance, can be rendered less effective by the use of certain medications, such as those used as part of medication-assisted therapy.

Therefore, patients need to discuss their usage of analytical hypnotherapy with their healthcare professional, who can advise them on the most effective way to include this sort of treatment in their already established strategy. Analytical hypnotherapy has the potential to be an effective component of an individual's comprehensive treatment strategy when it is administered under the supervision of a qualified professional and with all necessary safety measures taken.

It is crucial to keep in mind that although analytical hypnotherapy is a useful treatment option for many mental health conditions, it might not be the best choice for everyone. Therefore, if you are thinking of using analytical hypnotherapy as a possible method of treatment, it is necessary for you to first discuss your options with your primary care physician. Your primary care physician or another qualified medical professional can assist you in determining whether or not the treatment might be useful given the specifics of your case. In addition to this, they will be able to offer guidance on the appropriate preventative steps to take so that you can get the most out of the treatment. If analytical hypnotherapy is not the right course of treatment for you, your physician may recommend other methods of care instead.

Who Should Not Undergo Analytical Hypnotherapy?

Although analytical hypnotherapy may be a successful method of treatment for a variety of mental health conditions, not everyone is a good candidate for this approach. The following are some examples of people who should not submit themselves to this kind of treatment:

1. Individuals who refuse to consider the possibility of hypnosis

Those individuals who are resistant to the concept of hypnosis make up the first category of persons who should not participate in analytical hypnotherapy. A well-trained therapist can guide a patient into the relaxed and focused state known as hypnosis. Patients are often awake and able to hear and respond to the hypnotherapist while they are under the influence of hypnosis; but, following treatment, patients sometimes have problems remembering what took place during the hypnosis session.

2. Individuals who are diagnosed with a mental illness

Those who are diagnosed with a mental disease make up the second category of individuals who should not participate in analytical hypnotherapy. Depression, anxiety, bipolar disorder, schizophrenia, and eating disorders are all examples of diseases that might fall under the umbrella of mental illness. Because of these situations, it may be more challenging for a person to respond favorably to hypnosis, and the experience of hypnosis itself may even be more unsettling for them.

3. Individuals who are visibly impaired due to the effects of alcohol or other drugs

Those who are intoxicated by alcohol or drugs are the third kind of individuals who should not participate in analytical hypnotherapy since it might compromise their safety. It is much more challenging for a person to respond favorably to hypnosis if they are under the influence of alcohol or drugs, which might impede their capacity to concentrate and focus. In addition, the use of alcoholic beverages or illegal narcotics might make it more challenging for a person to recall what transpired during the session after the fact.

4. Those who have been through a tragic experience

Those who have been through a traumatic event make up the fourth category of individuals who should not participate in analytical hypnotherapy. Abuse acts of violence or even natural catastrophes can all be examples of traumatic occurrences. Because of the psychological anguish that can be caused by these occurrences, it may be difficult for a person to relax and concentrate when under hypnosis. In addition, traumatic experiences might make it more challenging for a person to place their confidence in their therapist and adhere to the recommendations they provide.

5. Individuals who have been diagnosed with Alzheimer's disease or dementia

Those who are diagnosed with dementia or Alzheimer's disease make up the fifth category of individuals who should not submit themselves to analytical hypnotherapy. Memory loss is a common symptom of Alzheimer's disease and dementia, two conditions that can make it challenging for a person to recall what transpired during a session after it has concluded. In addition, having one of these diseases might make it challenging for a person to focus and concentrate when under the influence of hypnosis.

6. People who have seizure disorders

People who suffer from seizure problems make up the sixth category of individuals who should not submit themselves to analytical hypnotherapy. People who suffer from seizure disorders are more likely to lose consciousness under hypnosis, which can put them in a very perilous situation. In addition, having a seizure disease might make it challenging for a person to remember what transpired during the session after it has been over.

Before ever contemplating analytical hypnotherapy, you are required to have a conversation with your primary care provider about whether any of the aforementioned conditions apply to you. They will be able to evaluate your situation and offer guidance about whether or not this method of treatment is appropriate for you. If analytical hypnotherapy is not the best course of treatment, they could also recommend other approaches.

When evaluating different types of treatment, you should always make sure that protecting your health and avoiding harm to yourself are your top priorities. Before beginning analytical hypnotherapy, you must get any questions or concerns addressed by speaking with your primary care physician.

Analytical Hypnotherapy vs. Psychoanalysis

Both analytical hypnotherapy and psychoanalysis are types of psychotherapy that are centered on assisting individuals in better comprehending the nature of their mental health conditions, building coping mechanisms, and making constructive adjustments to their lifestyles. Both of these methods include talking things through with a therapist in a setting that is confidential and free from criticism. But which of these is the best? To have a better understanding of this, let's compare and contrast these two distinct approaches to psychotherapy.

The goal of analytical hypnotherapy is to assist patients in achieving deeper levels of insight into the psychological challenges they are facing by utilizing a variety of techniques, including hypnosis, relaxation techniques, meditation, and visualization. During trance states, patients undergoing analytical hypnotherapy are encouraged to investigate the contents of their subconscious brains.

Because of this, they can obtain a deeper knowledge of the prior events that may be influencing how they behave and how they feel about life at present. In addition to this, patients who undergo analytical hypnotherapy are assisted in recognizing self-defeating patterns of thought and behavior that are no longer beneficial to them. People who are dealing with issues such as anxiety, depression, addiction, and post-traumatic stress disorder may find that this sort of treatment is particularly helpful (PTSD).

Traditional conversation therapy, dream analysis, and free association are all components of the psychoanalytic approach, which is often known as psychoanalysis. Its goal is to assist patients in uncovering memories or sentiments that have been buried deep inside their subconscious and may be the source of emotional anguish or behavioral issues. For the patient to be able to break away from self-destructive routines or obsessive behaviors, the purpose of this sort of therapy is to provide the patient with the ability to acquire insight into his or her mental processes. Psychoanalysis is frequently utilized in the treatment of mental health conditions such as depression, anxiety disorders, and phobias.

Your unique circumstances and personal preferences are ultimately the most important factors to consider when determining the style of psychotherapy that will best meet your requirements. Analytical hypnotherapy is a fantastic method to reach deeper levels of insight, although psychoanalysis may be more beneficial if you need help understanding how your ideas and feelings impact your daily life.

Analytical hypnosis is a great approach to gaining deeper levels of insight. If you are not sure which method could be most effective for you, it is in your best interest to contact a trained therapist who can offer guidance that is adapted precisely to the circumstances of your case. No matter whatever path you decide to take, one thing is certain: if you want to regain control of your mental health, you need to start by seeking professional assistance.

Conclusion

Analytical Hypnotherapy is an effective method for individuals who are interested in delving into the depths of their subconscious mind and gaining a deeper understanding of mental health concerns. Hypnosis, relaxation strategies, meditation, and visualization are all components of this type of psychotherapy, which is designed to assist patients in achieving greater levels of self-awareness and effecting good changes in their life. A trained therapist can assist you in evaluating your situation and give guidance on whether or not this form of treatment is appropriate for you, even if it may not be appropriate for everyone. No matter the path you decide to take, getting professional assistance is a necessary step in the process of taking charge of your mental health.

We hope that this introduction to analytical hypnotherapy has provided you with some helpful information to get you started on the path to improved mental health and well-being.

Keep in mind that before making any decisions about your health, you should always discuss them with your primary care physician. It is important to keep in mind that analytical hypnotherapy is not intended to serve as a replacement for professional medical advice or treatment. You must have a conversation on the potential benefits of this type of therapy for your mental health plan with your primary care physician or another appropriately trained mental health provider. I wish you the best of success and warn you to be careful!

FAQ About Analytical Hypnotherapy

1. What is Analytical Hypnotherapy?

Analytical Hypnotherapy is a type of therapy that uses hypnosis to treat a variety of psychological disorders. The goal of analytical hypnotherapy is to help the client understand and resolve the root cause of their problem. This type of therapy can be used to treat conditions such as anxiety, depression, phobias, and addictions.

2. How does Analytical Hypnotherapy work?

During analytical hypnotherapy, the therapist will guide the client into a state of relaxation known as hypnosis. Once in this state, the therapist will help the client to access memories and emotions that may be causing their problem. The therapist will then work with the client to resolve these issues.

3. What are the benefits of Analytical Hypnotherapy?

There are many benefits of analytical hypnotherapy, including improved mental health, reduced stress levels, and improved relationships. Additionally, this type of therapy can also help to improve physical health by reducing pain levels and improving sleep quality.

4. Is Analytical Hypnotherapy safe?

Yes, analytical hypnotherapy is considered to be a safe and effective treatment for a variety of psychological disorders. However, it is important to work with a licensed and experienced therapist to ensure safety and efficacy.

5. How long does Analytical Hypnotherapy take?

The length of treatment will vary depending on the individual and the severity of their condition. However, most people will require between 6-12 sessions to achieve desired results.

6. How much does Analytical Hypnotherapy cost?

The cost of analytical hypnotherapy will vary depending on the therapist and the length of treatment required. However, most therapists charge between $100-$200 per session.

References and Helpful Links

Analytical Hypnotherapy. 17 July 2021, https://hypnotc.com/analytical-hypnotherapy/.

Analytical Hypnotherapy | Hypnoanalysis - Hypnotherapy Directory. https://www.hypnotherapy-directory.org.uk/approach/hypnoanalysis.html. Accessed 26 Feb. 2023.

Analytical Hypnotherapy Using Hypnosis – The Surrey Hypnotherapy Clinic.https://www.surrey-hypnotherapy.com/articles/analytical-hypnotherapy/. Accessed 26 Feb. 2023.

Dublin, iWeb Design and Development and Ruth. "Hypnoanalysis Is a Regression Therapy. The Idea Is That We Seek to Find and Remove the Root Cause of the Anxiety or Emotional State Associated with a Traumatic Event from the Past." Ruth Allen Hypnotherapy, 29 May 2017, https://www.ruthallen.ie/aspects-of-hypnoanalysis/.

"Hypnosis for Anxiety: Procedure, Benefits, and More." Healthline, 17 Jan. 2018, https://www.healthline.com/health/hypnosis-for-anxiety.

Kroger, William S. Clinical and Experimental Hypnosis in Medicine, Dentistry, and Psychology. Rev. 2nd ed, Lippincott Williams & Wilkins, 2008.

Weitzenhoffer, André M. The Practice of Hypnotism. 2nd ed, John Wiley & Sons, 2000. Open WorldCat, http://books.google.com/books?id=IchrAAAAMAAJ.

"What Is Analytical Hypnotherapy." Hypnotherapy for Health, http://hypnotherapyforhealth.ie/what-is-analytical-hypnotherapy/. Accessed 26 Feb. 2023.

www.ingramcontent.com/pod-product-compliance
Lightning Source LLC
LaVergne TN
LVHW012037060526
838201LV00061B/4660